MEAL PLANNER

This planner belongs to ______________________________

STUDIO
AIZ

HELLO!

We hope you love your new Meal Planner! Our planner has been thoughtfully designed to help you organise, plan and simplify your weekly meals.

Stuck for meal inspiration? Try striking up conversations with your community, family or friends to see what's on their menu - sometimes a simple conversation can spark inspiration! Pinterest is also one of our favourite sources for new recipes and meal planning ideas.

Still unsure what to cook? Don't worry, we've made a short list of some of our favourite dishes which you might want to add into your planner to try!

- Zucchini Slice
- Prawn Tacos
- Spinach and Ricotta Cannelloni
- San Choy Bow Lettuce Wraps
- Chicken Burgers
- Mushroom Risotto
- Salmon Rice Bowl
- Chorizo and Broccolli Pasta

Enjoy!

WEEKLY MENU

MONDAY

TUESDAY

WEDNESDAY

Notes

THURSDAY

FRIDAY

SATURDAY

SUNDAY

Shopping List

WEEKLY MENU

MONDAY

TUESDAY

WEDNESDAY

Notes

THURSDAY

FRIDAY

SATURDAY

SUNDAY

Shopping List

WEEKLY MENU

MONDAY

TUESDAY

WEDNESDAY

Notes

THURSDAY

FRIDAY

SATURDAY

SUNDAY

Shopping List

WEEKLY MENU

MONDAY

TUESDAY

WEDNESDAY

Notes

THURSDAY

FRIDAY

SATURDAY

SUNDAY

Shopping List

WEEKLY MENU

MONDAY

TUESDAY

WEDNESDAY

Notes

THURSDAY

FRIDAY

SATURDAY

SUNDAY

Shopping List

WEEKLY MENU

MONDAY

TUESDAY

WEDNESDAY

Notes

THURSDAY

FRIDAY

SATURDAY

SUNDAY

Shopping List

WEEKLY MENU

MONDAY

TUESDAY

WEDNESDAY

Notes

THURSDAY

FRIDAY

SATURDAY

SUNDAY

Shopping List

WEEKLY MENU

MONDAY

TUESDAY

WEDNESDAY

Notes

THURSDAY

FRIDAY

SATURDAY

SUNDAY

Shopping List

WEEKLY MENU

MONDAY

TUESDAY

WEDNESDAY

Notes

THURSDAY

FRIDAY

SATURDAY

SUNDAY

Shopping List

WEEKLY MENU

MONDAY

TUESDAY

WEDNESDAY

Notes

THURSDAY

FRIDAY

SATURDAY

SUNDAY

Shopping List

WEEKLY MENU

MONDAY

TUESDAY

WEDNESDAY

Notes

THURSDAY

FRIDAY

SATURDAY

SUNDAY

Shopping List

WEEKLY MENU

MONDAY

TUESDAY

WEDNESDAY

Notes

THURSDAY

FRIDAY

SATURDAY

SUNDAY

Shopping List

WEEKLY MENU

MONDAY

TUESDAY

WEDNESDAY

Notes

THURSDAY

FRIDAY

SATURDAY

SUNDAY

Shopping List

WEEKLY MENU

MONDAY

TUESDAY

WEDNESDAY

Notes

THURSDAY

FRIDAY

SATURDAY

SUNDAY

Shopping List

WEEKLY MENU

MONDAY

TUESDAY

WEDNESDAY

Notes

THURSDAY

FRIDAY

SATURDAY

SUNDAY

Shopping List

WEEKLY MENU

MONDAY

TUESDAY

WEDNESDAY

Notes

THURSDAY

FRIDAY

SATURDAY

SUNDAY

Shopping List

WEEKLY MENU

MONDAY

TUESDAY

WEDNESDAY

Notes

THURSDAY

FRIDAY

SATURDAY

SUNDAY

Shopping List

WEEKLY MENU

MONDAY

TUESDAY

WEDNESDAY

Notes

THURSDAY

FRIDAY

SATURDAY

SUNDAY

Shopping List

WEEKLY MENU

MONDAY

TUESDAY

WEDNESDAY

Notes

THURSDAY

FRIDAY

SATURDAY

SUNDAY

Shopping List

WEEKLY MENU

MONDAY

TUESDAY

WEDNESDAY

Notes

THURSDAY

FRIDAY

SATURDAY

SUNDAY

Shopping List

WEEKLY MENU

MONDAY

TUESDAY

WEDNESDAY

Notes

THURSDAY

FRIDAY

SATURDAY

SUNDAY

Shopping List

WEEKLY MENU

MONDAY

TUESDAY

WEDNESDAY

Notes

THURSDAY

FRIDAY

SATURDAY

SUNDAY

Shopping List

WEEKLY MENU

MONDAY

TUESDAY

WEDNESDAY

Notes

THURSDAY

FRIDAY

SATURDAY

SUNDAY

Shopping List

WEEKLY MENU

MONDAY

TUESDAY

WEDNESDAY

Notes

THURSDAY

FRIDAY

SATURDAY

SUNDAY

Shopping List

WEEKLY MENU

MONDAY

TUESDAY

WEDNESDAY

Notes

THURSDAY

FRIDAY

SATURDAY

SUNDAY

Shopping List

WEEKLY MENU

MONDAY

TUESDAY

WEDNESDAY

Notes

THURSDAY

FRIDAY

SATURDAY

SUNDAY

Shopping List

WEEKLY MENU

MONDAY

TUESDAY

WEDNESDAY

Notes

THURSDAY

FRIDAY

SATURDAY

SUNDAY

Shopping List

WEEKLY MENU

MONDAY

TUESDAY

WEDNESDAY

Notes

THURSDAY

FRIDAY

SATURDAY

SUNDAY

Shopping List

WEEKLY MENU

MONDAY

TUESDAY

WEDNESDAY

Notes

THURSDAY

FRIDAY

SATURDAY

SUNDAY

Shopping List

WEEKLY MENU

MONDAY

TUESDAY

WEDNESDAY

Notes

THURSDAY

FRIDAY

SATURDAY

SUNDAY

Shopping List

WEEKLY MENU

MONDAY

TUESDAY

WEDNESDAY

Notes

THURSDAY

FRIDAY

SATURDAY

SUNDAY

Shopping List

WEEKLY MENU

MONDAY

TUESDAY

WEDNESDAY

Notes

THURSDAY

FRIDAY

SATURDAY

SUNDAY

Shopping List

WEEKLY MENU

MONDAY

TUESDAY

WEDNESDAY

Notes

THURSDAY

FRIDAY

SATURDAY

SUNDAY

Shopping List

WEEKLY MENU

MONDAY

TUESDAY

WEDNESDAY

Notes

THURSDAY

FRIDAY

SATURDAY

SUNDAY

Shopping List

WEEKLY MENU

MONDAY

TUESDAY

WEDNESDAY

Notes

THURSDAY

FRIDAY

SATURDAY

SUNDAY

Shopping List

WEEKLY MENU

MONDAY

TUESDAY

WEDNESDAY

Notes

THURSDAY

FRIDAY

SATURDAY

SUNDAY

Shopping List

WEEKLY MENU

MONDAY

TUESDAY

WEDNESDAY

Notes

THURSDAY

FRIDAY

SATURDAY

SUNDAY

Shopping List

WEEKLY MENU

MONDAY

TUESDAY

WEDNESDAY

Notes

THURSDAY

FRIDAY

SATURDAY

SUNDAY

Shopping List

WEEKLY MENU

MONDAY

TUESDAY

WEDNESDAY

Notes

THURSDAY

FRIDAY

SATURDAY

SUNDAY

Shopping List

WEEKLY MENU

MONDAY

TUESDAY

WEDNESDAY

Notes

THURSDAY

FRIDAY

SATURDAY

SUNDAY

Shopping List

WEEKLY MENU

MONDAY

TUESDAY

WEDNESDAY

Notes

THURSDAY

FRIDAY

SATURDAY

SUNDAY

Shopping List

WEEKLY MENU

MONDAY

TUESDAY

WEDNESDAY

Notes

THURSDAY

FRIDAY

SATURDAY

SUNDAY

Shopping List

WEEKLY MENU

MONDAY

TUESDAY

WEDNESDAY

Notes

THURSDAY

FRIDAY

SATURDAY

SUNDAY

Shopping List

WEEKLY MENU

MONDAY

TUESDAY

WEDNESDAY

Notes

THURSDAY

FRIDAY

SATURDAY

SUNDAY

Shopping List

WEEKLY MENU

MONDAY

TUESDAY

WEDNESDAY

Notes

THURSDAY

FRIDAY

SATURDAY

SUNDAY

Shopping List

WEEKLY MENU

MONDAY

TUESDAY

WEDNESDAY

Notes

THURSDAY

FRIDAY

SATURDAY

SUNDAY

Shopping List

WEEKLY MENU

MONDAY

TUESDAY

WEDNESDAY

Notes

THURSDAY

FRIDAY

SATURDAY

SUNDAY

Shopping List

WEEKLY MENU

MONDAY

TUESDAY

WEDNESDAY

Notes

THURSDAY

FRIDAY

SATURDAY

SUNDAY

Shopping List

WEEKLY MENU

MONDAY

TUESDAY

WEDNESDAY

Notes

THURSDAY

FRIDAY

SATURDAY

SUNDAY

Shopping List

WEEKLY MENU

MONDAY

TUESDAY

WEDNESDAY

Notes

THURSDAY

FRIDAY

SATURDAY

SUNDAY

Shopping List

WEEKLY MENU

MONDAY

TUESDAY

WEDNESDAY

Notes

THURSDAY

FRIDAY

SATURDAY

SUNDAY

Shopping List

WEEKLY MENU

MONDAY

TUESDAY

WEDNESDAY

Notes

THURSDAY

FRIDAY

SATURDAY

SUNDAY

Shopping List

WEEKLY MENU

MONDAY

TUESDAY

WEDNESDAY

Notes

THURSDAY

FRIDAY

SATURDAY

SUNDAY

Shopping List

Made in the USA
Monee, IL
05 November 2026

67374719R00063